Pegan Diet

The Complete And Simple Recipe Book For Starting And
Maintaining A Healthy Lifestyle, With Immediate Effects
On The Body And Mind

I0083582

(The Comprehensive Introduction To The Vegan Diet)

Clarence Madden

TABLE OF CONTENT

Combining The Vegan And Paleo Diets To Create The Pegan Diet

Dairy and eggs are excluded from the vegan diet due to their animal origin. Veganism, as defined by avoiding as much harm as possible to sentient beings, is a method of existing in harmony with the environment. Vegans also avoid animal-derived products in their daily lives, as they do not consume them and do not include them in their diets. The vegan lifestyle excludes products such as leather, wool, silk, pearls, and beeswax that are derived from or exploit animals in some manner.

Ethical vegans have long extolled the health advantages of consuming only plant-based foods. Vegan diets that are well-planned include above-average amounts of fruits and vegetables, as well as high fiber and low saturated fat. Additionally, there is no cholesterol ingested.

Cholesterol, a sterol produced by the liver and found in all body cells, is present in all animal products. The body generates enough waxy substance for it to function normally, despite the fact that waxy substance is necessary for life. Too much cholesterol is harmful because it can accumulate between the layers of artery walls, forcing the heart to work harder to circulate blood. There is evidence that vegans are more likely to suffer from some of today's most prevalent health problems, such as type 2 diabetes, cardiovascular disease, obesity, and certain types of cancer, possibly due to their lack of cholesterol intake.

Vegan Diet Disadvantages

Noting that you must eliminate all animal products from your diet in order to consume enough protein is essential. Therefore, vegan diets may be deficient in protein, calcium, vitamin B-12, folate, and omega-3 fatty acids. Organic and sustainably grown foods are permitted, thereby reducing the likelihood of nutritional deficiencies.

In a vegan diet, white bread, white pasta, and white sugar are all examples of refined carbohydrates. Some vegan foods, such as artificial additives, refined oils, and processed foods, are inflammatory because they are not derived from animals. The Pegan diet discourages the consumption of inflammatory foods, which have been linked to obesity and disease.

In Reference To The Paleo Diet?

The modern Paleo diet closely resembles the diet of our pre-agricultural ancestors. Cavemen utilized hunting and gathering as part of their Paleo diet. Paleo dieters with contemporary lifestyles no longer have to forage for sustenance in forests, fields, and streams. There are only a few facts about primitive foods that you must know.

The Paleo diet is becoming increasingly popular among those seeking a healthier lifestyle. This diet excludes processed foods and refined sugars, as well as carbohydrates and dairy, in order to achieve a lean and muscular physique.

In addition, the Paleo diet is believed to have numerous health benefits, including increased energy levels and a reduced risk for diseases such as diabetes, heart disease, obesity, and cancer.

Paleo Diet Disadvantages

Vegetarians and vegans frequently find it difficult to adhere to Paleo diets due to their reliance on animal proteins. Paleo permits some individuals to pile their plates with meat while conveniently ignoring vegetation.

In addition, by excluding grains, potatoes, and beans, this diet drastically diminishes the availability of fiber-rich foods. Consequently, you may consume less fiber, which is essential for digestive health.

Additionally, it can be difficult to adhere to the Paleo diet over the long term, particularly when traveling. Included in both the Paleo and Pegan diets are potatoes, gluten-free grains, legumes, peas, and unprocessed soy. Pegan diets offer greater variety and adaptability, making them more appropriate for those who wish to permanently alter their lifestyles.

Section Four

 How should legumes, whole grains, nuts, and seeds be consumed?

Eating the appropriate varieties of beans, whole grains, nuts, and seeds is essential to a healthy and balanced diet. Here are some suggestions for integrating these foods into your diet in a nutritious and healthy manner:

• Regularly integrate a variety of beans, such as black beans, kidney beans, lentils, and chickpeas, into your diet.

• Choose whole grains such as quinoa, brown rice, oats, and barley instead of refined grains such as white rice and pasta. Nuts and seeds are an excellent source of healthful fats and protein, but they can be high in calories, so consume them in moderation.

Consider soaking or sprouting your legumes, grains, nuts, and seeds before cooking or consuming them to improve their digestibility and nutritional value.

The key is to choose high-quality, unprocessed versions of these foods and to incorporate them into your diet in a manner that suits your needs and preferences.

SECOND CHAPTER

Consume beef as medication

The Pegan diet is a combination of the paleo and vegan diets, so it emphasizes whole, unprocessed foods and plant-based foods. Eating meat as medicine in the context of the Pegan diet refers to the notion that consuming high-quality, nutrient-dense meats can have a favorable effect on one's health. This may involve enhancing digestive health, boosting the immune system, and supplying essential nutrients that promote overall health and wellness. Notably, the Pegan diet continues to emphasize plant-based foods as the foundation of a healthy diet, and meat should be ingested in moderation as part of a balanced, whole-foods-based diet.

SECOND PART

How to be selective regarding chicken, eggs, and fish?

When following the Pegan diet, it is essential to choose antibiotic- and hormone-free poultry, eggs, and fish of the highest quality. These are some guidelines for selecting these foods:

Look for poultry that is organic, free-range, and reared humanely. Avoid conventionally raised poultry, which may contain antibiotics and hormones.

Eggs: Select organic, free-range, and humanely raised eggs. These eggs are more likely to be nutrient-dense and devoid of potentially harmful additives.

Choose wild-caught fish over farmed fish because wild-caught fish is typically higher in nutrients and lower in environmental contaminants. Avoid eating mercury-rich fish, such as swordfish and shark.

In addition to these recommendations, it is essential to consume a diversity of poultry, eggs, and fish to ensure a balanced diet. This may involve consuming a variety of fish, such as salmon, tuna, and cod, as well as selecting various poultry cuts, such as chicken, turkey, and duck.

SECTION SEVEN

Consume fats with each meal In the context of the Pegan diet, eating fat with every meal indicates that you should consume a healthful fat source with each meal. This is due to the fact that healthy fats are an essential component of a balanced diet and can provide a variety of health advantages, including supporting heart health, enhancing brain function, and promoting healthy skin and hair. Nuts, seeds, avocados, and olive oil are all examples of foods that contain healthy lipids. Not all fats are created equal, however, and it is essential to choose healthy fats that are unprocessed and free of Tran's fats and other unhealthy additives. Fats should be ingested in moderation and should not be the primary focus of the Pegan diet.

EIGHT

Avoid dairy

One of the essential principles of the Pegan diet is to consume as little dairy as possible.

You can avoid dairy on the Pegan diet by employing the following strategies:

• Select plant-based substitutes for dairy products, such as almond milk, coconut milk, and soy milk. These alternatives are readily available in most grocery stores and can be used to replace dairy in a variety of recipes.

• Use dairy-free spreads and condiments in lieu of butter and other dairy-based spreads, such as hummus, avocado, and nut butters.

• Experiment with dairy-free culinary and baking techniques, such as replacing cow's milk and butter in recipes with nut milks and oils.

• Carefully read food labels to avoid concealed sources of dairy in processed foods like breads, cereals, and snacks.

• When dining out, inquire about dairy-free menu options and make special requests for dishes to be prepared without dairy ingredients.

It is also essential to remember that each individual is unique and that what works for one person may not work for another. If you are uncertain about how to avoid dairy on the Pegan diet, or if you have concerns about your health, it is always advisable to consult with a healthcare provider or registered dietician who can offer personalized advice and support.

NINE

Feed like a regenetarian A regenetarian is a vegetarian who occasionally consumes humanely reared, sustainable animal products. If you wish to consume a Pegan diet as a regenetarian, consider the following advice.

• Prioritize consuming a diversity of whole, unprocessed plant-based foods, including fruits, vegetables, nuts, seeds, and whole grains. These nutrients should constitute the bulk of your diet.

• Select humanely raised, sustainable animal products such as grass-fed beef, free-range poultry, and wild-caught salmon, and consume them in moderation.

• Steer clear of processed and refined foods, as well as additives and preservatives.

• Carefully read food labels and select only those that are free of antibiotics, hormones, and other harmful compounds.

• Be mindful of your portion sizes and strive for a balanced diet that provides your body with the nutrients it requires without excessive consumption of any one food type.

Importantly, the Pegan diet is a flexible and individualized approach to food, and the specific guidelines for a regenetarian on the Pegan diet may vary based on your personal preferences and health objectives. If you are uncertain about how to consume as a regenetarian on the Pegan diet, or if you have any health concerns, it is best to consult with a healthcare provider or registered dietician who can provide personalized advice and support.

Your Gut And Immune System

You will be surprised to learn how much impact the digestive system has on the entire body. Unhesitatingly, we require additional pounds of food sources to be introduced directly into our gastrointestinal system multiple times per day. The digestive system is in charge.

Our capacity to convert the food we consume directly into fuel so that it can be absorbed and deliver various types of supplements. This will thus eliminate potentially hazardous substances from the body daily.

Consuming to Promote Digestive Health

Many of us have at one time or another considered discussing the microbiome.

Currently, many aspects of our wellbeing and health, such as longevity and weight loss, can be degraded by our waste. As Hippocrates asserted, "all diseases begin in the digestive system," the statement is true. While the science behind understanding the microbiome is not at the expected level, experts in utilitarian medicine have routinely dealt with a wide range of persistent diseases, including chemical awkwardness, weight concerns, headaches, immune system disease, skin issues, malignant growth cells, cardiovascular infection, diabetes, disposition issues, sensitivities, and so forth. According to a specific study, it has been confirmed that a waste transfer can reduce the signs of chemical imbalance by 50%.

From this, it follows that the microbiome is likely the primary health regulator. In actuality, you will be astonished to learn that there are more than 100 trillion microbiomes in your stomach alone, which is nearly multiple times your DNA and multiple times the number of cells in your body. Similarly, our microbiome contains more than three million microbial genomes.

A third to half of the multitude of particles that remain in our blood originate from microbial metabolites, which are associated with virtually every interaction in our science, including brain science, the immune system, hormonal specialists, and qualities, among others. Our intestinal system microorganisms also provide us with essential nutrients such as biotin and vitamin K.

Nevertheless, our intestinal microbiome is not in the same condition as it once was.

Today, we are all too familiar with absurd medications, lifestyle choices, and food sources. We all consume a processed diet that is high in artificial additives, carbohydrates, and sugar, but to our dismay, roughly 70% of plants are sprayed with the microbiome-destroying herbicide glyphosate. Our diet is deficient in polyphenols and prebiotic filaments, both of which are required for the development of beneficial microorganisms. In addition, we take a great deal of stomach-damaging anti-inflammatory drugs, corrosive blockers, and anti-microbial medications such as steroids, hormonal specialists, and Advil. From then on, we can include the impurities from the air, food, and water. Unfortunately, our body degenerates into a place filled with disease-causing agents and devoid of recovery agents. Inadequate food choices can lead to expansion, which is likely one of the primary causes of obesity and also persistent disease.

Under a one-cell-thin stratum of the stomach lining, approximately 60 percent of the invulnerable framework exists in the intestinal tract. When subjected to severe treatment, this cell layer will unquestionably promote a damaged stomach, allowing microbial toxins, microorganisms, and food proteins to "leak" into the circulatory system. As the scientific community evolves, researchers and clinical experts are gaining a deeper understanding of the relationship between digestive dysbiosis and persistent illness. In fact, my personal experience left me terrified. Around twenty-five years ago, mercury damage to my gastrointestinal microbiome was so severe that I developed diarrhea, abdominal swelling, and irritable bowel syndrome. I have finally been able to eliminate mercury from my system and recover my intestines. Clearly, this was not the story's conclusion.

Prior to a few decades, the quality of focal points began to deteriorate. My initial trench was treated with the antibiotic clindamycin, which led to the development of a fatal infection in my intestines known as C. Diff, which kills approximately 30,000 individuals annually. My body was in agony around-the-clock, and there were also additional symptoms and manifestations such as nausea, fever, loose intestines, bloody stools, etc.

My gastrointestinal structure was in shambles! This continued for the subsequent five months, and I am currently unable to concentrate on my work. I also began taking high doses of the steroid prednisone in a misguided effort to get better, but it was ineffective.

Thankfully, I began utilizing the principles of utilitarian medicine as well as repairing my digestive system and recovering its function.

standard capability. The scientific investigation behind the microbiome has progressed to such a degree that I was able to construct a novel method to treat and prevent gastrointestinal issues.

My colitis disappeared within three weeks after I began to engage in it directly. I altered my eating habits with the aid of various beneficial prescriptions. My method worked exceptionally well, and I am now able to treat every easily overlooked detail, including guiding meetings, irritable inside, and provoking gastrointestinal disease.

I started imagining my internal to be a solid and regulated nursery for the recuperation of my damaged digestive tract, which is the source of numerous persistent and incendiary diseases. It even helped me with excessive weight.

As soon as I imagined my digestive system as a nursery, I began utilizing three practices to cultivate a robust and balanced interior garden:

These ingredients are used to produce processed food sources that the American public is compensated for by the Food Stamp program. If a food company begins to fund a sustenance study, it is 50 times more likely that the study will demonstrate the food's benefit. Now that you have a thorough understanding of how the food industry operates, it is crucial that you choose an optimal diet. A pegan diet, as the name suggests, is a type of diet plan that adheres to the principles of both the paleo diet and the vegetarian diet. The Paleolithic era (more than 2.6 million years ago) was a time when meat, fish, vegetables, fruits, and seeds were readily available.

1. Consider over-the-counter drugs and foods as weeds. Therefore, the primary step is to eliminate the following food types from your diet: Steroids

Antibiotic medications, unless absolutely essential

carbohydrates, particularly sugar alcohols and artificial carbohydrates like high-fructose corn syrup.

Dairy, gluten, and any other sensitive food varieties, such as legumes, grains, and wheat, particularly if you have severe stomach dysbiosis.

Packaged or handled foods

Environmentally hazardous substances, such as maize, soy, and wheat; also avoid foods that have been sprayed with glyphosate Persistent pressure factors

Acid inhibitors

Anti-inflammatory drugs comparable to analgesics, such as naproxen (Aleve) and ibuprofen (Advil).

2. Add 'extraordinary annoyances' to your yard.

Once you have eradicated all of the harmful insects, it is time to introduce some beneficial insects to your garden, which include refined or aged food varieties such as:.

Unsweetened coconut yogurt Unpasteurized apple juice vinegar Regularly aged soy sauce Tofu (regularly aged) Tempeh (aged soy cake) Gluten-free tamari.

Miso.

Unsweetened kefir (ideally aged ewe or goat milk). Kimchi (aged vegetable or organic product) is fermented vegetables.

Sauerkraut that has developed naturally.

Next, you should take excellent care of your yard. You should consume foods that promote the development of solid microorganisms in the intestines. Comprises of sources of fiber- and prebiotic-rich foods. Clinical specialists recommend introducing prebiotic foods progressively if you have a low number of digestive bacteria. If you consume a large number of prebiotic food varieties at once, the symptoms may become worse.

Some exceptional examples of prebiotic dietary varieties

consist of Algae. Bananas and plantains that are unripe.

Polyphenol-rich foods, such as climate-friendly tea,

Pomegranate as well as cranberry.

Leeks, garlic, and additionally shallots Jerusalem artichokes Jicama start. Asparagus Artichokes Dandelion Apples are climate-friendly. The following dietary sources are rich in fiber:

Strawberries.

Pumpkin Spinach.

Olive oil just as olives Lentils.

Nuts as seeds specifically produced figs. Kale

Celery Cucumber.

Cabbage and broccoli sprouts.

Beans Avocadoes Berries.

If you are struggling with a severe case of intestinal dysbiosis, I would recommend a fantastic shake that will aid in the recovery of a wasteful digestive system. My colitis was cured in a short period of time. Due to thirty years of microbiome research, I concocted a drink that, in addition to healing my stomach, promoted the growth of healthy and balanced microorganisms such as Akkermansiamuciniphilus.

This particular microorganism maintains the physiological fluid and protects the layer to prevent a leaking digestive system. This microbe has been linked to cardiovascular disease, diabetes, obesity, immune system disorders, and even disease at low concentrations. If you do not have microorganisms in your framework, it is recommended that you avoid taking prebiotics. Flow research studies have demonstrated that Akkermansia thrives on the polyphenols found in green tea, pomegranate, and cranberry. In my case, polyphenols are the foundation for my inner yard. These micronutrients both nourish "incredible bugs" and rid my body of harmful microorganisms. Since I began experiencing this effect, I have been recommending the recipe for this shake to all of my family members and friends. When all else failed, this shake assisted me in treating my persistent condition. Additionally, it can be used to strengthen the intestine.

Here are the necessary ingredients for this smoothie.

A measurement of collagen powder.

A piece of your preferred high-potency probiotic (I used Xymogen's ProbioMax 350 DF).

A teaspoon of matcha climate-friendly tea powder, one tablespoon of concentrated cranberry juice, and one spoonful of concentrated pomegranate juice. One measure of acacia fiber.

An inside look at SBI Protect by NuMedicaImmunoG PRP. All you have to do is incorporate this assortment of ingredients with water to make a drink.

There is no doubt that practitioners of alternative medicine will be experts on digestive health. It makes no difference if you have a large amount of shock mercury in your system or are suffering from a parasite or infectious/bacterial overgrowth. A utilitarian medicine expert will examine your stomach wellbeing and health by analyzing your stool form, taking breath tests to look for an excess of negative irritants, and conducting food affectability tests in order to provide you with reasonable recuperation strategies and modified eating regimens. The vast majority of these specialists also offer instructive meetings, whether you choose to attend in-person or through online communication.

Consumables for the Immune System.

The vast majority of us regularly forget that we have a resistant framework, recalling them only when something goes wrong, for example, when we get a flaw. Imagine the problems if our resistant framework only existed for the initial two or three weeks of the winter season. However, this framework is continuously at work to keep our bodies healthy, well-adjusted, and functional by fending off the unrelenting pressure of pathogenic organisms such as viruses and bacteria.

Yes, the body's immune system is adaptive, which means that there is always a possibility of something failing, ranging from minor irritations such as the common cold to immune system disorders such as Type-1 diabetes. Eventually, there will be a microorganism that will overcome your body's immune system and make you ill.

Fortunately, there are a number of things you can do to ensure that your body's immune system continues to function normally for as long as possible; most of them do not involve medication. It has been determined that a paleo diet is sufficient to maintain the health of your body's immune system. This diet will reduce the stress that modern toxins have on your immune system, allowing it to focus on preventing infections such as the flu instead of wasting time with gluten in your bloodstream. When coupled with a healthy diet and sufficient rest, the body is constantly energized and prepared to deal with any type of antigen without the need for medication.

How exactly does the immune system function?

All organisms that cause infections, including microorganisms, infections, and parasites. Our body must eliminate antigens and other organisms from everything we imbibe, consume, contact, and ingest. If the person who contacted the handle before you has/had strep throat, then streptococcus may be transmitted to you.

Microorganisms have become a significant problem for you.

Thankfully, our body is equipped with a high-tech device that aids in warding off microbes; if not, we would not have been healthy. The invulnerable framework is the first line of defense; an adaptable response is required for any potential threat. This includes the actual barriers to disease, such as the epidermis, as well as bodily fluid film layers for internal defense, such as the coating of the digestive system. This implies that the streptococcus organisms on the door handle must first enter the body before they can kill you. This severe inventory will be an ideal entry point for strep microbes due to the invulnerable framework.

Inside, the opposition framework will continue to protect you with the aid of nebulous protection tools such as expanding, which is a flexible form of safe criticism. Expanding will produce a real deterrent and release related synthetic compounds to entice phagocytes, a type of body-dwelling cells that will destroy intruders. While expanding may receive a great deal of negative press, particularly in the paleosphere, it is not entirely dangerous. Assuming it becomes a recurring problem, this is truly awful news.

Even if the microorganisms are able to breach this barrier, they will still be required to navigate the flexible safe framework. While the conventional immune system offers a one-size-fits-all approach, the adaptable immune system will provide antigen-specific responses. The intrinsic body invulnerability framework is largely determined by the qualities you inherit from your parents. In contrast, the individualized immune system will acquire immunity to a variety of infections that may have previously infected you. Although the response time is substantially longer, it is unquestionably more reliable.

White platelets, also known as lymphocytes, perform the most important role in a versatile immune system. They are formed in the bone marrow and divided into two major types: B cells (B lymphocytes) and T cells (T lymphocytes).

The B cells generate various types of antibodies. B lymphocytes will remember streptococcus from a previous occasion.

Microorganisms also produce antibodies in a single second when strep throat is present.

Antibodies are extraordinary, but you must eliminate the microorganisms to achieve excellence. There are two types of T cells: the Helper T and the Awesome T. Paleo as well as immunity.

Most types of diets contribute to immune system problems. A paleo diet will aid in the prevention and treatment of such conditions, including less prominent immune system issues such as psoriasis and skin inflammation. A paleo diet routine can also help strengthen the immune system by reducing the number of antigenic irritants such as influenza and colds.

This is a stricter version of the paleo diet, in which nightshade vegetables and eggs are eliminated. Additionally, you can reintroduce a few food sources after the conclusion of the starter diet.

In addition to eradicating stomach poisonous aggravations, a paleo diet includes food varieties that heal the stomach by restoring a healthy population of intestinal microorganisms. There are a few naturally fermented food varieties, for example, kefir, kimchi, and sauerkraut, that help repopulate beneficial microorganisms in the stomach, shield the stomach-related divider surface from a specific type of microorganisms, and diminish the harm of antibiotics. Experts have found that probiotics can aid individuals with Crohn's disease and hypersensitivities. A low-carb diet can also eradicate microbial overgrowth problems such as

SIBO, which frequently causes digestive dysbiosis.

This does not imply that a zero-sugar diet is essential for immunity, particularly for those without digestive tract plant issues such as SIBO. A ketogenic diet will starve the defenseless microorganisms, and there are also microorganisms that prefer ketones to sucrose. The immune system requires sugar to fend off foreign invaders; however, a persistent no-carb diet will unquestionably diminish the body's ability to respond to them.

Sugar is also required to maintain the membrane cell lining on the stomach lining, which is one of the primary actual antimicrobials that protect the intestinal tract from infection.

Certainly, this may be somewhat frustrating for you: should you choose a diet where ketosis can help treat the excess of microorganisms and increase the resistance of certain microbes, or one where the consumption of starch will promote the growth of beneficial microorganisms and increase their resistance? the resistance of various microorganisms? Fortunately, there are advantages to both types of diets, which can only be achieved by cycling sugar consumption.

For instance, you can practice intermittent fasting, which will provide you with the benefits of ketosis without requiring you to eliminate carbohydrates from your diet. In addition to providing you with the benefits of both a low-carb and a moderate-carb diet, consuming safe carbohydrates in moderation will supply your body with sugar when you are not fasting.

In addition, the nutrient content of your diet plays an important role in preserving a healthy immune system. Extreme deficiency in any one minor component can have observable effects on an invulnerable element, which is extremely common in developing nations.

Numerous individuals suffer from a variety of less severe deficiencies; this interaction between them can impair the normal presentation of the resistant trait.

From the foregoing, it is normal for you to seek out various types of valuable Zinc or Vitamin C levels. However, consuming a healthy diet will ensure that your body's micronutrient levels are optimal.

In addition to diet, there are a number of non-dietary factors that can contribute to the development of high blood pressure. It will absolutely do wonders for your immune system!

m

What Should You Know About The Vegan Diet?

A pegan diet is a combination of the paleo and vegan diets, which seek to provide a sustainable and healthy balanced approach to eating. The diet emphasizes whole, unadulterated, nutrient-dense plant-based foods. In addition, it promotes the ingestion of healthy fats, such as those found in nuts, seeds, avocados, and certain types of fish.

When deciding what to consume on a vegan diet, it is best to prioritize nutrient-rich whole foods. Fruits and vegetables should make up the majority of the diet, along with nutritious proteins and fats. The focus is on proteins derived from plants, such as legumes, grains, and seeds. Also advocated are healthy fats, such as those found in olive oil and avocados.

Avoid eating processed foods, refined carbohydrates, and grains. Small quantities of dairy and eggs are permissible, but the majority of the diet should consist of plant-based foods.

The pegan diet also promotes healthy lifestyle habits, such as receiving sufficient exercise and rest. In addition, the diet encourages mindful dining, which involves being aware of how the food makes you feel and how much you consume.

The pegan diet is a balanced eating regimen that emphasizes whole, unprocessed, plant-based foods. It encourages the consumption of healthy fats, plant-based proteins, mindful eating, and other healthy lifestyle practices.

The best method for beginners to begin the vegan diet is to focus on whole, unprocessed foods. Start with minor adjustments and gradually add more plant-based foods to your diet. The most essential thing is to listen to your body and observe how various foods affect your mood.

With perseverance and fortitude, you can begin to experience the benefits of the vegan diet.

This page was left intentionally vacant

Advantages of the Vegan Diet

The Pegan diet combines the finest aspects of the Paleo and vegan diets to create a balanced, healthy lifestyle. The diet emphasizes whole, unadulterated foods and places restrictions on sugar, grains, legumes, and dairy. The Pegan diet offers numerous benefits for novices, including improved digestion, weight loss, and enhanced health.

Improved digestion is one of the primary benefits of the Pegan diet for novices. The diet is abundant in fiber-rich vegetables, fruits, nuts, and seeds, which aids in maintaining a healthy digestive system. In addition, the Pegan diet excludes common allergens, such as dairy and gluten, which can cause digestive problems in some individuals.

The Pegan diet is renowned for its ability to reduce blood sugar levels and inflammation in the body. This is largely attributable to the diet's low-glycemic, high-fiber content, which regulates blood sugar levels and reduces inflammation. In addition, the Pegan diet is abundant in healthy lipids, which can support healthy cholesterol levels and offer long-term cardiovascular benefits.

Overall, the Pegan diet is an excellent option for beginners seeking to achieve their weight loss and health objectives. The diet is well-balanced, nutritious, and simple to adhere to, making it an excellent option for those just beginning their health voyage.

Weight loss is another advantage of the Pegan diet for novices. Since the diet emphasizes whole, unprocessed foods and restricts sugar and simple carbohydrates, it is inherently low in calories and can aid in weight loss. In addition, the diet is rich in healthy fats, which can help stave off appetite and promote satiety.

Last but not least, the Pegan diet can also enhance overall health. Vitamins, minerals, and antioxidants are abundant in the diet, which can support a healthy immune system. In addition, the diet is abundant in healthful fats, which can reduce inflammation and improve cardiovascular health.

The Pegan diet is an excellent option for beginners seeking to lose weight and enhance their health. The diet is well-

49

balanced, nutritious, and simple to adhere to, making it an excellent option for those just beginning their health voyage.

This page was left intentionally vacant

Beverages Approved by Pegan

Beverages that are Pegan-approved contain natural, low-sugar ingredients and are devoid of dairy, added sugars, and refined grains. These beverages typically consist of water, unsweetened coffee and tea, coconut milk, nut milk, and kombucha.

Water is the most essential of all pegan-approved beverages, as it serves to flush out toxins, increase energy, and hydrate the body. Both unsweetened tea and coffee are excellent options because they contain antioxidants and stimulate the metabolism. Coconut milk and nut milks are rich in healthful fats, vitamins, and minerals, and can be substituted for dairy in smoothies, lattes, and other recipes. Kombucha is a fermented beverage that is probiotic-rich and can aid in digestion.

Regardless of the type of beverage selected, it is essential that it does not contain added sugars or refined grains. In addition, the ingredients should be fresh, organic, and free of preservatives and artificial additives. By adhering to these guidelines, individuals can experience a variety of pegan-approved beverages without jeopardizing their health.

The pegan diet is a great method to maintain a healthy lifestyle and includes a variety of delicious and nutrient-rich beverages.

Foods on the Pegan Diet

The Pegan diet combines the Paleo and Vegan diets. It promotes whole, unprocessed foods, moderate dairy consumption, and the avoidance of cereals, legumes, and processed foods.

Breakfast: Begin the day with a green smoothie prepared with spinach, kale, carrots, apples, and berries. Add almonds, seeds, or nut butter for protein.

Make a large salad with greens, tomatoes, bell peppers, cucumbers, and avocado for lunch. Dress the salad with a homemade vinaigrette. Add stewed sweet potatoes, roasted vegetables, and protein such as grilled chicken, tofu, or tempeh.

Snack on some raw fruits and vegetables, a sprinkling of nuts and seeds, or a piece of fresh fruit.

Have a serving of roasted vegetables, including broccoli, cauliflower, mushrooms, and bell peppers, for dinner. For whole cereals, add cooked quinoa, millet, or buckwheat, and for protein, add grilled chicken, tofu, or tempeh.

Banana ice cream will satisfy your sweet appetite as a dessert. Simply combine frozen bananas and a few teaspoons of almond extract in a blender until creamy. Add a few nuts or dark chocolate chunks for garnish.

These are a few suggestions for a vegan diet. With a little ingenuity, you can devise a variety of delectable and nutritious dishes.

Food to Avoid on Pegan Diet

A pegan diet incorporates elements of the paleo and vegan diets. It excludes refined and processed foods, dairy, legumes, cereals, and added sugars. It emphasizes consuming whole, unprocessed, plant-based, nutrient-dense foods.

These are some of the foods to avoid on a vegan diet:

Refined sugars are not only a source of empty calories, but they also cause blood sugar levels to rise. Avoid refined sugar in all of its forms, including white sugar, high-fructose corn syrup, and artificial stimulants.

Dairy products are high in saturated fat and cholesterol, which can contribute to a variety of health issues. Choose plant-based alternatives to milk and cheese instead.

Processed foods are typically high in unhealthy lipids, sodium, and sugar. Avoid all processed foods, such as chips and pastries.

Legumes can be difficult to assimilate and can stimulate inflammation. Choose instead other plant-based proteins such as almonds, seeds, and tempeh.

5. Refined cereals: Refined grains are devoid of nutrients and can lead to blood sugar spikes. Instead, opt for whole grains and pseudo-grains such as quinoa, buckwheat, and amaranth.

Alcohol: Alcohol contains no nutritional value and can cause a variety of health problems. Avoid it or consume no more than one drink per day.

7. Artificial sweeteners: Artificial sweeteners are frequently laden with chemicals and can have adverse health

effects. Choose natural sweeteners like honey, maple syrup, and dates instead.

By avoiding these substances, a healthy and balanced vegan diet can be maintained.

2.1 Cauliflower Fritters with Hummus

Prep Time: 15 mins

Cook Time: 15 mins

Servings: 4

Ingredients:

*   2 (15 oz) cans chickpeas, divided
*   2 1/2 tbsp olive oil, divided, plus more for frying
*   1 cup onion, chopped, about 1/2 a small onion
*   2 tbsp garlic, minced
*   2 cups cauliflower, cut into small pieces, about 1/2 a large head
*   1/2 tsp salt
*   Black pepper
*   Topping:
*   Hummus, of choice
*   Green onion, diced

Directions:

1.   Preheat the oven to 400 degrees Fahrenheit. 1 can chickpeas, rinsed and drained, placed on a paper towel to dry completely.

2. Place the chickpeas in a large mixing bowl, discard any loose skins, and toss with 1 tbsp olive oil. Spread the chickpeas on a large baking sheet and season with salt and pepper.

3. Bake for 20 minutes, then toss and bake for another 5-10 minutes, or until crisp.

4. After the chickpeas have been roasted, transfer them to a large food processor and process until they are broken down and crumbled - don't overprocess them and turn them into flour; you want some texture. Fill a small bowl halfway with the mixture and put it aside.

5. Add the remaining 1 1/2 tbsp olive oil to a large pan over medium-high heat. When the pan is hot, add the onion and garlic and sauté for 2 mins, or until the onion and garlic are softly golden brown.

6. After that, add the chopped cauliflower and cook for another 2 mins, or until golden.

7. Reduce to low heat and cover the pan; cook, frequently stirring, until the

cauliflower is fork-tender, and the onions are golden brown and caramelized about 3-5 mins.

8.   Transfer the cauliflower mixture to a food processor, drain and rinse the remaining can of chickpeas and add them, along with the salt and a touch of pepper, to the food processor.

9.   Stop to scrape down the sides as required until the mixture is smooth and begins to ball.

10.   Add 1/2 cup roasted chickpea crumbs to the cauliflower mixture in a large mixing bowl and stir until well combined.

11.   Pour enough oil into a large mixing bowl over medium heat to lightly coat the bottom of a large pan. Cook the patties in batches until golden brown, approximately 2-3 mins, then turn and cook the other side. Serve.

Nutrition: Calories: 333 Carbs: 45g Fat: 13g Protein: 14g

The Pegan Diet's Benefits

The Pegan Diet has three main categories of benefits: disease prevention, weight loss, and brain and gut health. Let's examine each of the three primary benefits of the Pegan Diet in greater depth:

Preventing Illness

Hypertension, type 2 diabetes, stroke, heart attacks, and other cardiovascular diseases, cancer, Alzheimer's disease, melancholy, Parkinson's disease, gallstones, and gallbladder disease can all be prevented with the Pegan Diet. How is this performed? The Pegan Diet contains a variety of high-fiber and antioxidant-rich fruits and vegetables. Antioxidants can help prevent a variety of diseases, including cancer, while fiber can help prevent fat absorption in the intestine.

Weight reduction

64

The Pegan Diet consists of approximately 50 percent low-calorie, nutrient-dense plant-based foods (fruits, vegetables, and whole cereals). The remaining fifty percent of the diet consists of plant-based proteins, healthy fats from nuts, seeds, salmon, and seafood, and low-fat dairy products. In brief, the Pegan Diet is more nutrient-dense than calorie-dense. Due to its minimal calorie density, it will never cause obesity or weight gain.

Adopting the Pegan Diet will help you achieve a healthy weight without resorting to extreme measures. This is due to the fact that the Pegan Diet contains more fiber than any other diet. Fiber makes you feel full and keeps you feeling full, so you do not need to consume as much food.

2) The Pegan Diet consists of an assortment of plant-based foods from which you can select those that are beneficial to you. For instance, if you

appreciate apples and oranges but dislike broccoli, you can choose between the two fruits with ease.

3) The Pegan Diet is designed specifically to help you expend more calories than other diets. This is due to the fact that it contains both lipids and carbohydrates. When the body metabolizes food for energy, heat is produced. The greater the presence of nutrients, the greater the heat produced, and consequently the greater the number of calories expended.

Cognitive and digestive health

The Pegan Diet will provide the necessary nutrients for optimal cognitive and gut health.

60% of the brain is constituted of fat. In two ways, the Pegan Diet will benefit your brain: It contains nuts, beans, legumes, and whole grains, all of which are excellent sources of vegetable protein and healthy fats; and it contains omega-3 fatty acids, which are essential for mental health.

The Pegan Diet can improve your memory and brain function in general; it can also improve your gut health, which promotes good digestion and the breakdown of undigested food in the intestines; it can reduce skin inflammation in acne patients and prevent eczema by interrupting the chain of inflammatory reactions in skin cells. How does it improve digestive health? The Pegan Diet includes soluble fiber (found in fruits, vegetables, nuts, legumes, and cereals in particular) and insoluble fiber (found in whole grains). The consumption of soluble fiber aids in the prevention of diverticulitis and diverticulitis. Insoluble fiber helps relieve constipation.

By decreasing intestinal permeability, the Pegan Diet can help prevent inflammatory bowel disease; it can also enhance bowel movements, treat diarrhea, and prevent colon cancer.

The Pegan Diet has been shown to aid in the healing of gastric ulcers, reduce the incidence of gallstones, and relieve irritating skin conditions including atopic dermatitis (eczema), urticaria (hives), and psoriasis.

The 75% Rule and Sugar Administration

What is the criterion for 75%?

The 75% Rule is a Pegan Diet recommendation indicating that 75% of one's meals should consist of vegetables.

It has been demonstrated that vegetable-rich diets have numerous health benefits, including weight loss and blood pressure reduction.

When will the rule be implemented?

The rule must be followed for the first three weeks of the vegan diet; after that, you may be able to progressively reduce or eliminate vegetables from your diet.

Suggestions for Planning: Plan your meals for the week in advance and ensure that each meal adheres to the Pegan Diet by emphasizing the combination of meat and vegetables.

Why Do I Need to Follow the 75% Rule?

This rule is intended to help you feel full, obtain all essential nutrients and vitamins, and maintain sufficient vitality throughout the day to remain active. By consuming a preponderance of plant-based foods and limiting your consumption of animal products, you will achieve more sustainable weight loss results than if you simply reduced your caloric intake.

How Should A Vegan Dietary Strategy Sugar?

In contrast, sugar is not always detrimental. The problem is that the overwhelming majority of individuals consume excessive quantities. Fortunately, vegetables and fruits contain naturally occurring sugars that are permissible on the Pegan Diet, as well as other nutrients that will keep your body satiated for hours.

Those with hyperglycemia should increase their consumption of sweet potatoes, carrots, and verdant green vegetables (broccoli and cauliflower's green florets). These have been shown to naturally balance blood sugar levels without causing medication-related side effects such as diabetes or an increased risk of cardiovascular disease.

Sugar is an illegal substance.

Consider the sensations you experience following sugar consumption. Do you ever experience fleeting energy that rapidly fades? Does sugar influence your feelings and actions? Consequently, sugar may be functioning as a stimulant for you. You may develop a dependency! The chemical reactions and reward centres of our brains become accustomed to sugar's effects on our bodies, and as a result, we crave it repeatedly despite being overweight or obese. The daily sugar intake limit for women is 100 calories (two tiny pieces of cake) and 150 calories of added sugar (one can of soda). Men should not exceed 150 calories per day from added carbohydrates (approximately one can of soda).

How Should the Least Harm Principle Be Applied?

Remember that the Pegan Diet is neither paleo nor vegan, but rather a combination of the two. This strategy is healthier than a conventional meat-only diet and more sustainable than a strict vegan diet.

The second stage is to reduce your carbon footprint by choosing organic meat, eggs, and produce whenever possible and avoiding processed foods.

The Peganism diet incorporates the Paleo and vegan diets. It is designed to maximize nutrition with the fewest conceivable sacrifices. For instance, a vegan may avoid consuming fish and chicken because of their animal origin, whereas a Paleo dieter may avoid eating potatoes and winter squash. Vegans and others who desire to maintain their current diet while obtaining the same health benefits as those following the Paleo diet may consider peganism.

How to Start

If you are considering undertaking the Pegan Diet, consider the following points:

Consult with your physician before beginning any diet.

Even if you're searching for a quick fix, make this diet a permanent change in your lifestyle.

Incorporate as much variety as possible into your diet by consuming foods from the different Pegan food groups.

Avoid processed foods and fast cuisine, and consume as little sugar as possible.

If your goal is to lose weight, you must consume the right number of calories for your requirements.

Remember that this diet is intended to be followed for an extended period of time.

Plan your meals meticulously and maintain a food journal to track the quantities you consume.

The Pegan Diet is a combination of two special diets - the Paleolithic and Ketogenic - and requires careful planning to be balanced and beneficial for the body. The following are some suggestions for getting started:

Consume a balanced diet consisting of at least 50 percent lean proteins, vegetables, and fruits from each category. Consume lean, fat-free sources of protein. The meats you should purchase are lean cuts of beef, poultry, turkey, and pork. In addition, seafood is an excellent source of protein. This includes salmon, shrimp, tuna, and anchovies, to name a few examples.

Consume a diet abundant in vegetables and fruits (each at 50 percent). Fruits and vegetables are essential for providing your body with the nutrients it requires to maintain good health. You should seek out vegetables such as spinach and kale that are green and verdant. Broccoli, bell peppers, tomatoes, onions, squash, and cabbage make excellent additions as well. Apples, cranberries, mangoes, and strawberries are all superb fruit alternatives.

Consume moderate amounts of lipids (25 percent). Healthy lipids are essential for fat loss and body maintenance. Healthy lipids include avocado, olive oil, nuts, fatty fish, and seeds.

Consume sufficient carbohydrates (25 percent). Carbohydrates are not the enemy of this diet; however, they must be ingested in moderation in order to prevent weight gain. Excellent carbohydrates include beans, legumes, quinoa, cereals, and whole grains such as brown rice and whole wheat. Sweet potatoes, which are rich in vitamins and minerals, can also be used as a source of carbohydrates.

Allow for time for exercise. It is not necessary to engage in strenuous exercise; a daily stroll will suffice. Consider incorporating yoga or Pilates into your routine for increased flexibility and strength.

Remind yourself to consume an adequate amount of water throughout the day. You must drink plenty of water throughout the day to maintain hydration. This will ensure adequate nutrient intake and may help you feel satisfied.

Avoid overstressing or overpressuring your body (no excessively lengthy workouts or hefty lifting).

Avoid processed foods at all costs; avoid anything with more than five listed ingredients on the label.

Sweet potato and black bean breakfast burrito with salsa:

Description: This tasty and satisfying breakfast burrito is filled with a flavorful and nutritious combination of sweet potatoes, black beans, and salsa, and it can be enjoyed hot or cold.

Preparation time: 10 minutes

Cook time: 15 minutes

Ingredients:

• 1 sweet potato, peeled and diced
• 1/2 cup black beans
• 1/4 cup salsa
• 1/4 cup shredded cheese
• 1 tortilla

Preparation:

• Preheat the oven to 400°F.

- Spread the sweet potato pieces on a baking sheet and roast for 15 minutes, or until they are tender and caramelized.
- Meanwhile, heat the black beans in a small saucepan over medium heat until they are hot.
- Warm the tortilla in a dry pan over medium heat until it is pliable.
- Spread the black beans, sweet potatoes, salsa, and cheese onto the tortilla.
- Fold the sides of the tortilla over the filling and roll it up tightly to form a burrito.
- Serve the burrito hot or wrap it in foil to enjoy as a grab-and-go breakfast.

Health Advantages Of The Vegan Diet

The Pegan diet has numerous advantages, with weight loss being the most significant. But there are others as well, and when they all work together, it not only helps drop the number on the scale, but also promotes clearer thinking and a healthier, happier existence overall.

Helps Efficiently The last word is not a joke: weight loss. According to scientific research, unused sugar and carbohydrates are promptly stored as fat. Healthy fats, a cornerstone of the Pegan diet, are not deposited as fat because they are not processed by the liver. In fact, the body prefers fat over carbohydrates and basic sugars as an energy source, at least over the long term. Therefore, unless you run marathons or exercise for hours, you will never burn off those stored calories from sugar and unhealthy carbohydrates. In addition, many individuals spend the entire day seated at a desk. However, the Pegan diet is not based solely on caloric intake and expenditure. It's more about the types and timing of calories consumed. It emphasizes the character of our food selections rather than their quantity. You heard correctly: There is no calorie counting! And it is effective. In the early stages of writing this book, when I followed my own advice more closely, I lost the last few pounds I had been attempting to lose for some time. And they have remained absent.

Have you ever had uncontrollable appetites for Ben & Jerry's ice cream, pizza at any time of day, bagels, bready sandwiches, or chocolate, chocolate, and more chocolate in any form? Prior to adopting a Paleo and then a Pegan lifestyle, these were my irrational cravings. These high-protein, low-carb, low- or no-sugar regimens are effective for a reason. Even in the form of an artificial sweetener, carbohydrates and sugar cause insulin levels to rise. If you consume carbohydrates or sugars frequently throughout the day, even in the form of foods that are considered by some to be healthful, such as orange juice, whole-wheat toast, or gluten-free pasta, insulin levels remain elevated even at night. This can result in insulin resistance in instances of prediabetes and type 2 diabetes. Carbohydrate consumption has addictive properties; it induces cravings for more and more carbohydrates (so don't excuse your lack of self-control). Like excessive alcohol consumption, excessive insulin can cause an obese liver. Double horrors.

Reduces Abdominal Fat and Preserves Lean Muscle: As we now know, consuming too many processed foods and not enough whole, fresh foods can result in chronic inflammation within the body. Chronic inflammation not only provides the groundwork for the development of potentially harmful diseases, but it also causes an increase in cortisol levels, which can induce a state of constant stress. This hormone imbalance results in the accumulation of visceral fat, which accumulates around major organs and enlarges waistlines. By emphasizing a colorful variety of fresh, whole foods in their purest form and limiting dairy, you can prevent these hormonal changes from reducing abdominal obesity. And, you predicted it, when you lose belly fat, you also lose weight. Adding even a small quantity of strength training to your routine will enhance the Pegan lifestyle's effectiveness. You will notice more muscle definition. Lean muscle mass consumes calories more efficiently throughout the day than abdominal fat. This is essential not only for weight loss, but also for weight maintenance once your objective has been reached.

Regulates Appetite: Excess insulin causes issues with appetite regulation by inhibiting leptin in the brain. You will feel famished even though your body has sufficient energy. By not worrying about calories and focusing on selecting high-quality, fresh, whole foods the majority of the time, you will notice that your body will naturally regulate your appetite whenever you settle down to a meal or consume food on the go. You will remember what true hunger feels like and be able to give your body only what it requires. When your ability to perceive satiety improves, you will likely eat less in general, which, you predicted it, results in greater weight loss!

Enhances Mental Clarity and Boosts Energy: Eliminating processed carbohydrates and added sugars will result in a life-altering energy boost. It was the case for me. Two factors result in this: The lack of sugar in your diet helps prevent erratic, emotional, addiction-like behaviors and cravings for unhealthy foods; additionally, by increasing our consumption of foods rich in omega-3 fatty acids, such as walnuts, avocados, grass-fed beef and butter, and low-mercury fish, we are actually sending energy to and nourishing the brain. Neurons desire fat; feeding them fat improves their firing rate. Recent research indicates that healthy fats are not only beneficial for cardiac health, but also for brain and nerve health. In addition to the mental clarity you will experience, consuming vegetables and other whole foods will provide you with more energy than you could have imagined.

As was the case with me, your total cholesterol level may rise after adopting a Pegan diet for an extended period of time. This is likely due to the increase in healthy cholesterol levels (HDLs), even if the levels of harmful cholesterol (LDLs) remain stable or, better yet, decrease. We now know that neither saturated fat nor eggs are the villains that they were once thought to be. However, processed foods and oils, in addition to sugar and processed carbohydrates, have been linked to elevated blood pressure and LDLs, which can lead to heart disease.

Low Glycemic burden: Nearly all diets aim to reduce the glycemic burden on the body. The Pegan diet effectively reduces and regulates glycemic levels. Reducing the amount of sugar, flour, and refined carbohydrates reduces glycemic index and diabetes risk.

Pllar for Pegan consuming 1. Stay clear of sugar: This pertains to both refined sugars and high-sugar foods such as fruit.

The regan diet uses a "75/25 plate" rule, which states that 75% of your plate should be low glycemic index (GI) vegetables and 25% should be protein, such as meat, nuts and seeds, cereals, or legumes.

3. Add fruit in moderation: Fruit is a healthy addition to a diet, but it is high in sugar and has a high glycemic index. People with diabetes or who struggle to lose or maintain a healthy weight should consume fruit in moderation and avoid it altogether. Berries with a low glycemic index are an exception and can be consumed in moderation.

4. Avoid retinoids, antibiotics, hormones, and GMO foods: The diet emphasizes eating natural, non-manufactured foods. The key is to consume foods that are as near to their natural state as possible.

Many fruits and grains, such as wheat and maize, that have been hybridized and modified to increase their sugar and starch content, as well as animals that have been given antibiotics and hormones, are neither healthy nor nutritious.

Include an abundance of healthy fats: A healthy diet includes nuts, seeds, avocados, oils such as walnut, avocado, and olive, and grass-fed dairy products such as butter and raw milk. These fats contain essential omega-3 fatty acids.

6. Avoid most vegetable, nut and seed oils: These oils are high in omega-6, making it challenging to maintain a healthy omega-3 to omega-6 ratio. A diet that is excessive in omega-6 fatty acids is inflammatory.

7. Choose dairu wiselu: Manu people are intolerant to dairy rrodusts. If these products induce digestive issues, you should avoid them. If there are no complications, the healthiest options are

grass-fed butter, heavy whipping cream, and raw sheep's milk.

Consider meat and animal byproducts as condiments: Meat and seafood are the best sources of protein, an essential nutrient for maintaining or gaining muscle mass.

9. Consume utanablu-raised, low-mersuru eafood: Smaller fish, such as salmon, sardines, herring, and anchovies, contribute high-quality protein and fat to the diet. Larger fish higher on the food chain have higher mercury and other toxic concentrations.

10. Avoid gluten: Approximately three-quarters of the world's population has varying degrees of gluten intolerance, which is not commonly recognized or treated. Even in individuals who are not gluten-intolerant, new research indicates that gluten can damage the intestines.

11. Consume gluten-free whole carbohydrates in moderation: Grains can be part of a healthy diet, but they are high in carbohydrates and contain few nutrients. Some healthier alternatives include wild rice, buckwheat, and quinoa.

12. Eat beans ossasionallu: Legume (lentils, soy, and bean) have a low ratio of protein to carbohydrate relative to animal protein and are high in starch. Theu are healthy additions to a diet in moderation, but those who have difficulty digesting them, are diabetic, or struggle to lose or maintain a healthy weight should avoid them.

13. Get evaluated to validate your diet: We all have different nutritional requirements and professional backgrounds. Nutritional deficiency or issues such as heavy metal toxicity can be helpful in determining optimal health.

What To Consume On A Vegan Diet

The Pegan diet emphasizes "healthy" food. This includes whole foods and foods that have undergone minimal processing.

Fruits and vegetables, especially those with a low carbohydrate content or glycemic index, such as broccoli, carrots, peas, and tomatoes.

Almonds, pistachios, and walnuts are seeds.

Seeds, including chia, flax, and pumpkin

Grass-feed meat such as beef, poultry, and pork.

Salmon, herring, and cod are high-fat, low-mercury fish.

Eggs

Gluten-free cereals, such as quinoa, brown rice, oatmeal, and amaranth (occasionally).

Eat more produce

The majority of your pegan diet should consist of vegetables and fruits, which should account for 75% of your total intake.

To minimize blood sugar response, you should prioritize low-glycemic index fruits and vegetables, such as berries and non-starchy vegetables.

Those who have achieved healthy blood sugar control prior to beginning their diet may consume a small quantity of starchy vegetables and sweet fruits.

Consume few processed lipids.

In this regimen, you should consume healthy fats from the following sources:

Olives and Avocados

Nuts: except peanuts

Coconut: Unrefined coconut oil is beneficial.

Omega3

except for refined seed oil

Legumes and Some whole cereals are ingestible.

Small amounts of gluten-free whole grains and legumes are permitted in the diet, despite the fact that the majority of grains and legumes are discouraged because they may impact blood sugar levels.

Cereal consumption per meal should not exceed 1/2 cup (125 grams), and legume consumption per day should not exceed 1 cup (75 grams).

The following cereals and legumes can be consumed:

Black rice, quinoa, amaranth, millet, thrush, and oats are grains.

Lentils, chickpeas, black beans, and pinto beans are legumes.

However, these foods should be restricted further for diabetics and those with other diseases that cause poor blood sugar control.

What to avoid on a vegan diet

Gluten and dairy are essential components of this diet. Additionally, you should avoid or limit the consumption of processed foods that contain additives to extend their expiration life.

These foods should be avoided on a vegan diet:

Bread, pasta, baked products, cereals, granola, and beer are examples of staple foods.

Cheese, yogurt, and milk

Lentils, beans, and peas are legumes.

Products containing pesticides

Any food containing artificial preservatives, colors, flavoring, or sweeteners

Is the Pegan diet beneficial to health?

No extensive research has been conducted on the health effects of a vegan diet.

But many people concur that a plant-based diet consisting of fruits and vegetables high in fiber and low in starch can improve overall health and reduce the risk of certain diseases. Several studies have demonstrated that plant-based diets can reduce weight and harmful cholesterol levels.

If you do not have any intolerances or health conditions (such as celiac disease), you are not required to avoid gluten. Long-term, its exclusion will make it difficult to adhere to a diet. In some instances, it can even deplete the body of nutrients. According to studies, incorporating whole grains and legumes into one's daily diet can enhance overall health.

Benefits of pegan diet

A Pegan diet can improve health in numerous ways.

The heavy emphasis on the consumption of fruits and vegetables may be its finest quality.

Fruits and vegetables are among the healthiest diets. They are abundant in fiber, vitamins, minerals, and plant compounds known to prevent disease, reduce oxidative stress, and reduce inflammation.

Additionally, the pegan diet emphasizes the heart-healthy, unsaturated fats found in salmon, nuts, seeds, and other plants.

In addition, a diet consisting primarily of whole foods and containing almost no ultra-processed foods is associated with an improvement in diet quality overall.

What Exactly Is a Pegan Det?

The "regan" diet is a hybrid that combines the raleo diet, which focuses on whole foods that were hunted or gathered, such as fruits, vegetables, meats, and nuts, with the vegan diet, in which you consume only plant-based foods.

The pegan diet combines concepts from the paleo and vegan diets on the premise that nutrient-dense, whole foods can reduce inflammation, maintain blood sugar levels, and promote overall health.

If you initially believed that being both paleo and vegan would be difficult, you're not alone.

The regan det is unique and has its own set of rules despite its appellation. Fasting is less restrictive than a raleo or vegan diet on its own.

Vegetables and fruits are prioritized, but small to moderate amounts of meat, certain fish, nuts, seeds, and legumes are also permitted.

Heavy rroseed sugars, ol, and cereals are discouraged, but permissible in very small quantities.

The regan diet is not intended to be a standard, short-term diet. Instead, it seeks to be more sustainable so that you can adhere to it indefinitely.

The combined sore characteristics of the pegan det are as follows:

1. Extremely low in glucose, meaning low in sugar, flour, and refined carbohydrates.

2. A diet rich in vegetables and fruits, with a focus on variety. At least 75% of meals should include fruits and vegetables.

3. Low in retidine, antibiotics, and hormones, as well as no or low levels of GMOs.

4. No shemsal, additives, preservatives, sucralose, monosodium glutamate (MSG), artificial sweeteners, or other "Franken Chemicals."

5. Rich in healthful fats, such as omega-3 fatty acids.

Adeuate rroten for arrhythmia control and muscle relaxation, particularly in the elderly.

Ideallu, liver, and fresh foods should comprise the majority of the diet.

8. Selecting utanablu-raised or grass-fed meats when consuming animal products.

Selecting fish with minimal levels of mersuru and toxins.

What You Should Remember

Since fruits, vegetables, and meat comprise the majority of the vegan diet, these foods are non-negotiable if you choose to adopt a vegan lifestyle. However, you may have to make individual decisions regarding how much you are willing to pay for non-GMO, shem-free produce and grass-fed meat.

Since the vegan diet limits or excludes rice, legumes, and grains, you will need to be extra vigilant about consuming the nutrients that these foods provide.

If you eliminate dairy products such as yogurt from your diet, you may need to increase your consumption of fermented foods such as kimchi in order to obtain gut-boosting probiotics. You may also include sardines, eggs, and an abundance of green leafy vegetables such as broccoli to replace some of the calcium and vitamin D you would normally obtain from milk.

What Can You Consume?

Unlike some diets, there are no rules regarding what to eat for breakfast, lunch, and dinner. It provides a general outline of dietary advice based on a number of basic criteria.

The main tenets of a vegan diet include eating foods with a low glycemic load; eating a lot of fruits, vegetables, nuts, and seeds (about three-quarters of your daily intake); eating grass-fed or sustainably raised meat when you do eat meat; avoiding sugar, additives, preservatives, and genetically modified organisms; and getting plenty of healthy fats.

Vegan Diet For Healthful And Long-Term Weight Loss

More and more people are attempting the Veggie Lover Diet, also known as the Plant-Based Diet, in an effort to shed unwanted pounds. In contrast to keto eat fewer carbs, which is difficult to maintain and not heart-healthy in the long run, the Vegetarian Diet is a whole-food plant-based eating plan that is healthy, practical, and offers immunity-boosting food varieties to keep your energy up and your defenses strong as you lose weight.

The Adele Diet, also known as the Sirtfood Diet, is featured in a number of online weight loss programs. (We attempted it and the results were as follows.) At that juncture, irregular fasting occurs. (Which also works if you consume substantial meals during the "on eating hours.")

Currently, more people are endeavoring to consume a plant-based diet than ever before: 23% of consumers are incorporating plant-based or vegetable-lover food sources into their diet: Since the height of the Coronavirus emergency, sales of plant-based meats have risen 35%, while sales of all vegetarian food sources have risen 90%. People need a diet that enables them to get in shape and stay healthy, and a vegetarian or plant-based "clean-eating" diet ensures both: In addition to consistent weight loss, solid resistance is exhibited during the process of getting in shape.

Robust Weight Loss, Less Fatty Kid Arrangement With Plant-Based Protein

The Vegetarian Diet and Plant-Based Diet are gaining popularity because they are more sustainable than other diets. In addition, it is largely consistent with its appearance. You avoid irritation-inducing animal products and consume plant-based whole food varieties that are low in oil, minimally cooked, and rich in fiber. Prepare yourself to have your consciousness blown. It functions.

However, there are two reasons why the Veggie lover Diet is so popular right now: One is that people are avoiding meat during the Coronavirus outbreak, and the other is that the Vegetarian Diet helps you get in shape and construct your immunity. It is also reasonable, sensible, and typical. There is nothing more regular than consuming a plant-based diet that is low in oils and calories.

The Veggie devotee Diet is by and large what it seems like: You consume enormous quantities of vegetables, natural products, fruits, cereals, nuts, and seeds. There is no purpose in counting carbohydrates, calories, or net carbs. You fill your plate with whole plant-based foods that are low in oil, barely cooked, and rich in fiber. If you can make it happen, it's a "Go!" If you need to seek for ingredients on a label and there are numerous, it is "Off limits!" This method of getting in shape is natural, instinctual, and practicable. If you lose 2 pounds per week, which is a healthy rate, you will have lost 12 pounds by the fourth of July.

The Veggie Lover Diet For Weight Loss Is Well-known During Coronavirus Season.

Why is the Veggie Lover Diet experiencing a resurgence? Primarily meat processing plants are still infested with Coronavirus, and just this week, Tyson was forced to shut down its largest pork facility after 555 of its employees tested positive for the infection. This implies that store network interferences will likely increase the price of meats, and consumers are concerned that meat could spread the disease, despite the absence of evidence that this has occurred.

Then, on the potential gain, the Vegetarian Diet is prevalent, allowing the calorie counter to load up on vegetables and fruits, grains, nuts, and seeds, in addition to the organic product - all food types that are rich in fiber, satiatingly filling, and provide a great deal of dietary protein. Listed below are the types of foods that contain the most protein, in all honesty. For most calorie counters, obtaining enough protein on a vegetarian diet begins with a bowl of oats and plant-based milk, which is about a quarter of the way there. There is an easy, low-calorie meal.

Why The Veggie Lover Diet Is Effective: Fiber Is A Distinct Advantage For Weight Watchers To Shed Fat

The greater the fiber content of supplemental food sources, the better they are. Fiber has received unfavorable criticism as a "controller" for individuals with constipation, but it is actually the "counter carb" when it comes to consuming high-quality food sources that stimulate weight loss. When diabetics are placed on a strict low-carb diet, they are instructed to seek out fiber because the fiber-to-carb ratio is more important than carbohydrates alone. This is why organic food, despite being higher in carbohydrates than vegetables, does not cause weight gain.

The fiber in the food you consume enables the body to absorb healthy nutrients while keeping glucose levels and insulin response under control. The lower your blood glucose level, the lower your insulin response, and the less your body is signaled to store excess energy as fat.

Due to the high fiber content of plant-based foods, the "net carb" effect provides all of the nutrients with fewer calories, carbohydrates, and undesirable fat than animal products or highly processed food sources. Therefore, the key to getting in shape on the Veggie lover Diet is selecting food sources that are as close to their natural state as possible. Whole plant-based food varieties, such as vegetables, organic products, vegetables, nuts, seeds, and grains, provide a solid combination of nutrients and minerals, proteins, and complex carbohydrates, allowing the dieter to feel satisfied and full, never hungry and deprived, and still lose weight.

At the point when your fat admission is low - no animal fat and negligible oils - your body will create prepared energy based on what has been stored in the body. You deplete glycogen first, and as anyone who has endured a 45-minute spin class or run likely knows, you switch your energy system when you run out of available stored energy in the muscles and liver, and then begin to consume fat stores and extract energy from capacity. The low-oil vegetarian diet is a natural way to stimulate your body to find energy from within, essentially revving up your machinery to copy fat faster.

Stay Healthy As You Lose Weight With Immunity-Boosting Vegetables and Natural Products

The Veggie Lover Diet is rich in vegetables and organic foods with resistance-enhancing properties. On the "list" of the Vegetarian Diet are all of the dietary sources that are known to help maintain normal immunity. Broccoli, mushrooms, peppers, and citrus are among the thirteen food types that offer the greatest resistance per bite.

The Veggie Lover Diet can help you achieve reasonable weight loss by limiting your consumption of prepared foods that are likely to be high in added sugar and fat, low in fiber, and full of added substances. While potato crisps are generally vegetarian, they do not qualify because they are processed. The same applies to Twizzlers and other packaged foods that are vegetarian because they do not contain animal products. To become more physically fit, you must consider, "If I can grow it, I can eat it." You have never witnessed a PopTart in a daycare.

When you consume the Veggie lover Diet, you become healthier because you avoid inflammation-inducing animal products and fill your plate with plant-based whole food varieties that are low in oil, clearly cooked, and rich in fiber. In addition, expect to be stunned. It functions. You can lose up to 2 to 3 pounds per week and maintain the loss by adhering to a vegetarian or plant-based diet.

Since you are opting for the combined benefits of the Paleo and Vegan diets, you stand to gain a great deal from adopting the Pegan diet. If weight loss were your primary concern, you would do well to eliminate grains and dairy from your daily diet. Consider that they are either refined or processed, both of which are unhealthy. If you find it difficult to completely abstain from them, at least during the initial stages, you may indulge occasionally.

Diabetes will hesitate to attack you if your diet is devoid of refined flours, sugar, and refined carbohydrates. Ultimately, the glycemic burden is too low for anything harmful to occur in the body. Add to this the fact that you consume healthful fats containing Omega-3 fatty acids, and you reduce your risk of cardiovascular disease even further. Even your cognitive function will be preserved as you age.

As stated previously, no diet is regarded complete without regular exercise or physical activity. Since you are accustomed to eating lean meat and fish, you can anticipate that your muscles will regain their fitness and strength as they eliminate excess fat and replace it with healthy protein.

Fresh fruits and vegetables are rich in essential minerals and micronutrients. Their phytonutrient content will ensure that your body remains healthy. Minerals and micronutrients cannot be created by the body; they must be obtained from outside sources. Additionally, your altered dietary habits prevent hazardous substances from entering your systems. They continue to be non-toxic.

Saving Cash While Being Pennywise

In many parts of the world, nutritious and organic foods are significantly more expensive than processed foods. The healthiest method to eat is to cook your food, which will require additional time for shopping and preparation. This is a luxury few working individuals can afford. Numerous individuals cannot afford to invest extra time and money. Especially not when inexpensive, delicious precooked dishes are readily available on every street corner.

This catastrophe is responsible for the prevalence of obesity, weight gain, inflammation, and other health problems. However, even when finances and time are limited, there are ways to make pegan a possibility.

A common misconception is that dining out is less expensive than cooking at home. When purchasing ingredients in abundance and not tipping a waiter, the same meal can be prepared for pennies. When you prepare meals at home, you eliminate the excess oils, sodium, and sugar that restaurants add to their dishes.

The best method to save money on vegan ingredients is to shop for groceries carefully. Buying fresh ingredients in bulk is a wonderful way to stretch their value. It is preferable to purchase items like sweet potatoes, rice, and culinary oils in bulk rather than in individual portions.

Purchasing dry legumes in quantity and rehydrating them yourself will also save money. When purchasing dry legumes in bags or cartons, you receive significantly more food for a lower price. It will last for weeks in a pantry and is environmentally favorable because it eliminates the need to continually buy cans. All that is required is to leave them overnight in water; the process is not at all time-consuming.

Meal preparation is an additional method to save money. When a busy and stressful day arrives, it can be extremely inconvenient to consider what we will consume. Cooking and cleaning additional dishes during a busy work week is not optimal. Instead of preparing on-site, many people wait in a drive-thru line. This is bad for your wallet and your health.

This issue can be avoided by preparing meals early in the week, such as on Sunday. You save time, money, and petrol.

Meal preparation is not as challenging as one might assume. Consider, for instance, Sunday supper. Why cook only one chicken breast when you can cook four? You are already controlling the stove and adding seasonings, so it requires no additional effort. Set aside the surplus for the following few days, and then repeat. There are four simple dinners that require no preparation and minimal additional effort. In addition, you did not have to dash to the store for additional ingredients or wait in line for a quick meal elsewhere.

Healthy food does not always resemble expensive grocery stores and oversold supplements. If you know what to search for, you can find nutritious food in virtually every supermarket. This is illustrated by frozen vegetables, which are ordinarily economical. Frozen vegetables and fruits are flash-frozen as soon as they are harvested, making them fresher than produce in the produce aisle.

Other vegetables, such as tinned tomatoes, are inexpensive and nutrient-dense. The cheapest grocery stores contain, among other inexpensive foods, oatmeal, brown rice, canned salmon, carrots, cabbage, and sweet potatoes.

When purchasing in volume, preparing meals in advance, and acquiring inexpensive vegetables, you spend significantly less than you would on junk food and processed foods. In addition, when you consume pegan, you avoid hundreds of health conditions caused by excessive consumption of carbohydrates, sugar, and processed food chemicals. In turn, you save thousands of dollars in medical costs associated with treating these preventable diseases.

Cooking at Home

Cooking at home saves money and produces far superior results than store-bought dishes. Cooking is a wonderful way to share nutritious food with loved ones, and it can even become a creative and enjoyable hobby.

On the other hand, eating out may appear healthful. Nonetheless, restaurants and rapid food establishments add ingredients you wouldn't add yourself. Many international chain restaurants reheat frozen ingredients in the microwave. These foods are preserved with preservatives and sodium to make them taste as delicious as fresh food. You would not dare add as much butter, sugar, and table salt to your own cuisine as restaurants do. Even if you order something that appears to be perfectly healthy, it is impossible to know precisely what the chef added to give it its flavor.

When cooking, you have complete control over what goes into your cuisine. You, and not someone else, decide what you place into your body. And the greatest part is that you can make delicious food without spending additional money.

In the following chapters, I will introduce you to fifty simple and delectable recipes that will inspire you and help you maintain a vegan diet. By utilizing these recipes, the guidelines and advice outlined in this chapter, and your newly acquired knowledge of nutrition, you will be successful on the vegan diet.

Distinct From Other Common Diets?

A Pegan diet can be thought of as a hybrid of various forms of diets. However, it remains distinct from the others. Learn how the Pegan diet is distinct from other prevalent diets.

Paleo

A paleo diet is, by definition, the belief that eating in the manner of our ancestors is optimal for human health. This diet contained limited quantities of nuts and seeds, healthy oils, organic foods, vegetables, and livestock. It permitted nothing artificial, dairy products, beans, potatoes, grains (including maize), and processed foods. Meats ingested are typically lean, and there would be no agricultural production of crops and grains. In general, grass-fed and natural food sources would make up the majority of the diet.

In contrast, a Pegan diet combines the finest aspects of the paleo and vegetarian diets. Therefore, you consume solid oils, natural products, vegetables, and proteins in smaller portions while avoiding added sugars, gluten, and dairy.

One of the greatest misinterpretations of a paleo diet is that the diet consists primarily of'meat'. Logic dictates that a diet consisting solely of meat would have been inconceivable for mountain folk. Huge creatures are difficult to capture, and a great deal of time would be devoted hunting them.

As a result, our ancestors began supplementing their diets with nutrient-dense foods such as almonds, vegetables, natural products, and vegetables.

However, this is where the similarities between a Pegan and paleo diet end. Due to the absence of gluten grains such as rice, maize, and oats on a paleo diet, getting in shape is significantly more difficult. This is because the absence of these foods adds a substantial number of extra calories. Due to the Pegan diet, you do not consume more than one serving of gluten per day.

Vegan

The only distinction between a vegan diet and a Pegan diet is that a vegan diet is entirely plant-based, whereas a Pegan diet must consist of at least 75% plants. A vegan diet is defined as a lifestyle that excludes all animal-based products, including those used for apparel, food, and other purposes. Therefore, a vegan diet excludes animal products such as dairy, eggs, and meats.

People choose a vegetarian diet for a variety of reasons, ranging from ecological to moral concerns. However, they may also be motivated by a desire to enhance health.

In contrast, a Pegan diet is virtually identical to a vegetarian diet. As opposed to consuming plant-based cuisines as side dishes, Pegans consume items derived from creatures. The main components of this diet are exclusively vegetarian.

In addition, a Pegan diet excludes dairy products.

According to the preceding, a vegan diet is very similar to a Pegan diet. In the case of a vegan diet, you exclude meat, poultry, and fish from your diet. Additionally, vegans exclude from their lifestyles and diets other animal-based products, such as honey and eggs, as well as any other products that contain animal byproducts, such as leather, mohair, cosmetics, etc. Animal-based products are permitted on a Pegan diet; however, they should make up no more than 25% of your menu; the remaining 75% must consist of plant-based foods.

 Vegetarian

Some individuals may choose a plant-based diet and avoid eating meat for a variety of reasons. By definition, a vegetarian diet excludes all foods derived from animals, including eggs, dairy products, fish, poultry, and meat. Similarly, a vegan diet excludes all animal-based foods, including salmon, fish, poultry, and meat. However, they are permitted to consume a few animal-based products, such as dairy.

When comparing a vegetarian diet to a vegan diet, there are numerous similarities. For instance, both diet types include plant-based nutrients.

However, this is where the similarities cease. On a Pegan diet, you are not permitted to consume dairy products such as margarine, milk, etc.

Furthermore, it is prohibited to polish cereals, whether they are whole or refined.

In contrast to the Pegan diet, you are not permitted to consume animal-based foods such as meat, eggs, and dairy products. However, this also depends on the type of vegan diet that you adhere to. For instance, a flexitarian diet, also known as a semi-vegetarian diet, permits the consumption of dairy products and eggs, as well as limited amounts of salmon, fish, poultry, and meat. The Pescatarian diet prohibits the consumption of poultry and red meat, but allows seafood, fish, dairy products, and eggs.

Keto

A Pegan diet and a ketogenic diet are both low-calorie plant-based diets; however, their emphasis is different. The ketogenic diet has a strong preference for plant-based foods, while the Pegan diet has a comparable preference for the paleo diet. While there are numerous similarities between the two, there are also significant distinctions.

Will Cole, a renowned beneficial clinical professional, developed the ketogenic diet. As a result of observing the efficacy of the ketogenic diet on his patients, he switched to consuming fewer calories. While some keto dieters consume a large deal of animal fats and products, Cole modified his diet so that fish was the primary source of animal protein.

Yes, it is possible to follow a vegetarian-only version of the ketogenic diet because the diet is defined by whether you are in healthy ketosis. In light of the hypothesis, it does not matter how you enter the ketosis state; you can enter ketosis with both low-quality and substantial foods.

Both types of regimens aim to control glucose levels and reduce irritation. The two weight loss programs avoid vegetables, grains, meat, and dairy products for the most part. The best aspect of these weight control plans is that the restrictions are lenient; neither of the projects are extreme or controversial. Moreover, the two types of regimens permit you to consume 'illegal' food varieties occasionally if it does not cause a problem. In general, you cannot fail with either of the two types of regimens.

DASH

The DASH diet, also known as the Dietary Approaches to Stop Hypertension, is a dietary plan designed to treat hypertension without the need for medication. In addition to preventing diabetes, stroke, coronary illness, malignant growth, and osteoporosis, this form of diet is also used to prevent conditions such as diabetes, stroke, coronary illness, and osteoporosis.

Comparable to the Mediterranean diet, the average DASH diet consists of nuts, poultry, fish, whole cereals, low-fat dairy, organic produce, and vegetables. In any event, this diet restricts sodium consumption to no more than 2,300 mg per day. Despite the fact that this diet does not cause weight loss, many individuals experience weight loss as a result of making healthier choices.

When compared to the Pegan diet, the two diets share numerous similarities. Natural products, vegetables, and animal-based products comprise a portion of your entrée. However, you must ensure that the meat is lean for the DASH diet, while eggs, poultry, and meat must be humanely raised, organic, and grass-fed for the Pegan diet. While nuts are included in both weight control programs, the Pegan diet excludes whole grains, in contrast to the DASH diet.

In addition, the Pegan diet prohibits dairy products, whereas the DASH diet permits a low-fat diet. The main difference between the two types of diets is the result – people who follow DASH diets frequently experience health issues such as elevated blood pressure, whereas the foods mentioned prevent such conditions.

Mediterranean Diet

There are not a great deal of differences between a Mediterranean diet and a vegan diet when compared closely. It has been reported that a Mediterranean diet offers numerous health benefits, ranging from reduced stress and weight loss to a decreased risk of chronic diseases and ailments.

Based on research, it has been determined that a Mediterranean diet, along with not smoking and daily exercise, will prevent 90% of Type-2 diabetes, 90% of coronary heart disease, and 7% of stroke. You should merely make food choices that are consistent with a traditional Mediterranean diet.

When comparing the Mediterranean diet to a vegan diet, you'll notice that both revolve around superior eating plans. The two dietary plans emphasize consuming more fruits and vegetables. A Mediterranean eating routine follows the guideline of the paleo diet of avoiding bundled or handled foods.

The main contrast between the two weight control plans is the nature of creature items; the meat should be field raised, wild, and natural. Moreover, a Pegan diet likewise wipes out refined food sources like bread and entire wheat. Dairy items are likewise kept away from in a Pegan diet.

In this section, you will learn about the nutritional characteristics of the vegetarian and Paleo diets, as well as the numerous advantages of the Pegan diet. Pegan cooking offers the simplest healthy components of these two dietary forces to be reckoned with, as well as countless medical benefits, such as enhancing your health, preventing disease, reducing stress, and boosting your vitality. In addition to all of the specific benefits of a vegan diet, it is also highly adaptable and simple to incorporate into your daily life. You have no difficulty locating ingredients or utilizing novel cooking equipment or techniques. Always determine how this way of life can enhance your well-being and prosperity.

The Vegan Diet

The vegetarian diet excludes all animal-derived products, including dairy and eggs. Vegetarian is a term that can be used to describe an entire lifestyle, one that avoids causing as much harm to sentient beings as possible. Not only do moral vegetarians exclude all animal products from their diet, but they also renounce the use of all products derived from animals in their general daily lives. Cowhide, fleece, silk, pearls, and beeswax are excluded from the vegetarian way of life, along with other animal-derived or animal-abusing products. Since vegetarians are ethical vegetarians, a well-rounded vegetarian diet is high in fiber, low in saturated fat, and includes a greater proportion of foods grown from the ground.

Additionally, no cholesterol is ingested. Cholesterol, a sterol produced by the liver and discovered in the body's cells, is present in all creature parts. Even though the waxy substance will last eternally, the body produces everything it needs to function properly. Burning a lot of cholesterol can be dangerous because it causes plaque to form between the layers of the conduit dividers, making the intestines work harder to transport blood.

Studies indicate that vegetarians have a lower risk of some of the most serious medical conditions, including type 2 diabetes, cardiovascular disease, obesity, and a few types of cancer, possibly due to the absence of cholesterol in their diet.

The present health-conscious global community recognized these benefits, and as a result, veganism has taken on a new form: the vegetarian for health reasons. Those who choose a plant-based diet typically adhere to similar dietary guidelines (no meat, no dairy, no eggs, and no animal-derived condiments). However, enhancing their health and decreasing their risk of infection is their driving force.

What Can Vegans Consume?

Contrary to popular belief, vegetarians can stock their refrigerators and pantries with a vast array of foods. Pasta, soup, tortillas, oat, bagels, potato crisps, and wafers are just a few of the "ordinary" foods that vegetarians can devour. Moreover, a growing number of companies are developing palatable vegetarian products.

Identifying whether an item is vegetarian is a very simple task. Consider: "Did this come from a living animal?" If the permissible response is "Yes," then the creature is not a vegetarian.

Shouldn't We Say Something About Fish?

Does fish originate from a sentient creature? As fish, lobsters, and prawns are all living creatures, fish is not vegetarian.

What Can Be Said Regarding Nectar?

Does nectar originate from an animal? Since nectar is produced by bumblebees, which are animals, it cannot be consumed by vegetarians.

Shouldn't We Say Something About Gelatin?

Does gelatin originate from an animal? Gelatin is derived from the decomposition of animal bones, tendons, and skin; therefore, it is not vegetarian-friendly.

Therefore, the vegetarian diet prohibits anything that comes from a living creature. It is not difficult to comprehend that a cheeseburger, macaroni, cheddar, or omelet should not be consumed, and it is similarly easy to comprehend that plates of mixed vegetables, spaghetti with marinara, and tofu over rice are all on the "Yes" list. However, the situation deteriorates when endeavoring to consume suitable food varieties, such as boxed, canned, and prepackaged dinners. Reading product labels is essential when practicing a vegetarian lifestyle. Regardless, as a general rule, even individuals who do not have dietary restrictions must acquire the ability to recognize names. It is crucial to comprehend what is occurring within your body.

Where Do Vegans Get Protein?

The most frequent query asked of vegetarians is "Where does one obtain protein?" There are numerous plant-based sources of protein, as well as animal products. All prevalent food types (natural products, fruits, vegetables, grains, legumes, nuts, and seeds) contain protein. Lentils, couscous, tofu, tempeh, quinoa, peanuts, sunflower seeds, cereal, almonds, whole wheat bread, dark beans, chickpeas, corn, peas, avocado, spinach, flaxseed, broccoli, brown rice, seitan, edamame, great northern beans, chia seeds, and artichokes are examples of plant-based protein sources.

What Are the Drawbacks of a Vegan Diet?

A vegetarian diet entails eliminating all animal products and meeting protein requirements through cereals and vegetables. Consequently, the vegetarian diet is frequently deficient in essential nutrients such as protein, calcium, vitamin B12, folate, and omega-3 unsaturated lipids.

The Pegan diet permits natural, commercially raised animal products, thereby preventing food shortages. On the vegetarian diet, numerous individuals consume refined carbohydrates, such as white bread, white macaroni, and white sugar. Certain fiery food sources, such as artificial sugars, refined oils, and processed foods, are also permitted on the vegetarian diet because they do not originate from animals. On the Pegan diet, these incendiary food varieties are severely weakened due to their association with obesity and illness.

The Paleolithic Diet

The Paleolithic period, also known as the Old Stone Age, spanned from the beginning of human existence (2.5 million years ago) to around 12,000 B.C.E. The Paleolithic diet lauds the food sources that were consumed during this time. Meats, poultry, fish, insects, eggs, mixed greens, organic products, berries, nuts, and seeds constituted the Paleolithic diet. Paleolithic individuals were expert trackers whose diet consisted solely of foods discovered in nature.

The modern Paleo adheres to the exact same pre-agriculture diet as his ancient ancestors. The Paleo diet is full of foods that could have been hunted and gathered by mountain folk. Those on a Paleo diet do not need to forage for sustenance in the forests, fields, and streams of modern society. It is simply a matter of comprehending the customs of various raw food types.

The Paleo diet is becoming increasingly popular among those who wish to maintain a healthier lifestyle. Since processed foods and refined sugars are avoided, and dairy and carbohydrates are depleted, this diet promotes a fit and robust body synthesis. In addition, it is widely acknowledged that the Paleo diet has numerous health benefits, including increased energy levels and a reduced risk of diseases such as diabetes, cardiovascular disease, obesity, and cancer.

What Can a Paleo Dieter Consume?

Paleolithic individuals lived off the land and consumed only natural foods. Due to necessity, they pursued and gathered their food varieties before cooking them over a fire while adhering to an extremely short-sighted lifestyle. To determine whether an object is Paleo, simply consider whether an early human would have needed to cook it. New meats, new vegetables, and new organic products have taken center stage in the current Paleo diet. The key is keeping it simple and consuming only food varieties that originate directly from the earth, neither processed nor artificial.

The Paleo diet prohibits dairy, cereals, vegetables, and potatoes, among other foods. No milk or cheddar. No bread or bagels. No legumes, beans, peas, or soy allowed. In addition, adhering to the Paleo diet entails avoiding refined sugars and refined vegetable oils.

Where Does Paleo Get Protein?

It is not difficult to determine where Paleo dieters obtain their protein: from animal products. Meat is a significant component of the Paleo diet. Paleo meats should preferably be grass-fed or wild wildlife.

Despite the fact that meats constitute a significant portion of the diet, it is recommended that you avoid high-fat meats; lean meats are preferable. Fish, poultry, and eggs are also valuable.

What Are the Negative Aspects of the Paleo Diet?

Due to its heavy emphasis on animal protein, the Paleo diet can be difficult for vegans and vegetarians to follow. Similarly, the Paleo diet permits nearly everyone to fill their dishes with meat while omitting vegetables.

In addition, the inclusion of grains, potatoes, and legumes limits the variety of fiber-containing foods permitted on this diet. This may result in a decreased intake of fiber, which is necessary for digestive health.

Similarly, the Paleo diet is truly restrictive and may be difficult to adhere to, particularly when traveling or dining out. The Pegan diet includes all Paleo-approved food sources and others, such as potatoes, gluten-free grains, legumes, peas, and natural forms of soy. This considers more variety and adaptability, making the Pegan diet more suitable for a long-term lifestyle change.

The Pegan Diet: The Best of Both Worlds

To enhance the health benefits of both the vegetarian and Paleo diets, the Pegan diet emphasizes the consumption of natural, whole food varieties. Sources of food that arrive in a container are not acceptable for vegans. In fact, an inordinate number of the food sources you will purchase will not have a food name.

You will likely find yourself perusing at the Dinnermarket's perimeter. This diet promotes the selection of privately derived, natural, and minimally farmed food sources. During your Pegan experience, you will prefer to investigate the business sectors of nearby ranchers or to purchase at Dinner markets with more extensive natural produce sections.

Typically, this is how life alters, increasing one's enthusiasm for high-quality food varieties and propelling them beyond their usual comfort zone. The Pegan diet promotes optimal health by reducing inflammation and regulating glucose. It is widely acknowledged that this lifestyle has numerous health benefits, including weight loss, increased energy levels, and a decreased risk of diseases such as diabetes, cardiovascular disease, adiposity, and cancer.

Tomato Soup With Italian Flavor

- 2 tsp. tomato paste
- 2 bay leaf
- salt
- pepper
- 4 stems basil
- 400 g tomatoes (5 tomatoes)
- 1 onion
- 4 cloves garlic
- 2 tbsp. olive oil
- 2 tsp. oregano
- 200 ml vegetable broth

1. Scald tomatoes in boiling water for 5-10 minutes, then rinse under cold water, peel, cut in half, and cube the pulp.
2. Peel and finely cut the onion and garlic. In a saucepan, heat 1 tablespoon of oil.
3. When the onions and garlic are transparent, steam them.

4. Toss in the oregano.
5. combine the tomatoes and tomato paste in a mixing bowl.
6. Add the bay leaf, salt, and pepper to the vegetable stock.
7. Bring the soup to a boil, then reduce to a low heat and cover for around 10-15 minutes.
8. Clean the basil by squeezing it dry. Create fine strips out of the leaves.
9. Remove the bay leaf from the soup, and puree it with a hand blender.

Porridge With Cinnamon And Coconut

Ingredients

- 2 tablespoon butter
- 2 and ½ teaspoon stevia
- 2 teaspoon cinnamon
- Salt to taste
- Toppings as blueberries
- 4 cups of water
- 2 cup 36% heavy cream
- 1 cup unsweetened dried coconut, shredded
- 4 tablespoons flaxseed meal

Directions

1. Add the listed ingredients to a small pot, mix well
2. Transfer pot to stove and place it over medium-low heat
3. Bring to mix to a slow boil

4. Stir well and remove the heat

5. Divide the mix into equal servings and let them sit for 15 to 20 minutes

6. Top with your desired toppings, and enjoy!

Hash Of Sweet Potato, Sausage, And Cauliflower

Ingredients:

- 2 teaspoon minced garlic
- 1 lbs. grass-fed ground pork
- 1 teaspoon chili powder
- ½ teaspoon ground cumin
- 2 tablespoon olive oil
- 4 medium sweet potatoes, peeled and chopped
- 2 cup chopped cauliflower florets
- 2 small yellow onion, chopped
- Salt and pepper to taste

Instructions:

1. Heat the oil in a large skillet over medium heat.
2. Add the sweet potato and sauté for 5-10 minutes until browned.
3. Stir in the cauliflower, onion and garlic.

4. Add the water then cover the skillet and steam the vegetables for 1-5 minutes.
5. Remove the lid and stir in the sausage, chili powder, cumin, salt and pepper.
6. Let the mixture cook for 5 to 10 minutes until the meat is browned.
7. Flip the hash and cook for another 10 to 20 minutes until the bottom is browned and the sweet potatoes are tender. Serve hot.

www.ingramcontent.com/pod-product-compliance
Lightning Source LLC
Chambersburg PA
CBHW060507030426
42337CB00015B/1777